Office Procedures
for the Dental Team

Office Procedures

for the Dental Team

BETTY LADLEY FINKBEINER, C.D.A., R.D.A., B.S., M.S.

Instructor-Coordinator, Dental Assisting Program,
Washtenaw Community College,
Ann Arbor, Michigan

JERRY CROWE PATT, B.S.

Instructor, Department of Secretarial Office Careers,
Washtenaw Community College,
Ann Arbor, Michigan

SECOND EDITION

with 260 *illustrations*

The C. V. Mosby Company

ST. LOUIS • TORONTO • PRINCETON   1985

A TRADITION OF PUBLISHING EXCELLENCE

Editor: Darlene Warfel
Assistant editor: Melba Steube
Manuscript editor: Maureen Stephens
Design: Suzanne Oberholtzer
Production: Judith Bamert, Barbara Merritt, Susan Trail

SECOND EDITION

Printed in the United States of America

The C.V. Mosby Company
11830 Westline Industrial Drive, St. Louis, Missouri 63146

Library of Congress Cataloging in Publication Data

Finkbeiner, Betty Ladley, 1939-
  Office procedures for the dental team.

  Includes bibliographies and index.
  1. Dental offices—Management.   2. Office procedures.
3. Dental teams.   I. Patt, Jerry Crowe, 1932-
II. Title.   [DNLM: 1. Dental Assistants.   2. Practice
Management, Dental.   WU 77 F4990]
RK58.F56 1985   651'.96176   84-11577
ISBN 0-8016-2817-2

C/VH/VH   9   8   7   6   5   03/C/301

To
our students
and to
the memory of
Joseph S. Ellis, D.D.S.

FOREWORD
from first edition

Inasmuch as the dental assisting profession continues to evolve to a higher level of sophistication, a textbook that encompasses all the duties of the business assistant had to be forthcoming. As a general practitioner for 25 years, I believe that this book has arrived. *Office Procedures for the Dental Team* covers the dental business office practice in its entirety. The book is exceptionally well thought out and includes valuable details and excellent illustrations.

The authors' diversified background provide a well-balanced distribution of information. One of them has had many years of experience in dental offices, while the other has had extensive training in the business field.

The book is designed to teach assistants at all levels. It can also serve as an excellent reference in all types of practices and can be a means for stimulating discussions during personnel sessions both in the classroom and in the office setting.

I am privileged to write this foreword, and I feel strongly that this long overdue textbook will do much to improve our dental care delivery system.

Robert L. Morrison, D.D.S., B.S.
General Practice
Las Vegas, Nevada

PREFACE

Over the past 10 years we have team-taught a dental office procedures course for dental assistants. During this time the modern dental office has expanded its utilization of dental auxiliaries, and the dental business office has been no exception to this advanced technology. In this revision we have continued to satisfy the needs of dental assistants and dental student about to establish a new practice as well as those dental assistants and dentists already in practice.

Keeping in mind the diverse background of our readers, we have maintained the objectives of our first edition and have expanded these objectives to reflect new technology and the need to have "hands on experience" before the actual activity in the dental business office. Therefore we have provided a comprehensive text that will accomplish the following objectives: (1) be understandable to all of our readers, (2) provide behavioral objectives for competency-based education that are augmented by the text material, (3) be a procedural textbook as well as a reference manual, (4) present authentic illustrations, (5) provide working experience using actual forms, (6) introduce automated technology into the dental business office, (7) emphasize the importance of the business assistant as a vital member of the dental health team, and (8) stress the importance of business technology and management in the dental office.

We have combined our own business and dental assisting experience with the experiences of practicing dentists and dental assistants in an effort to integrate these two dynamic professions. This second edition continues to touch only the tip of an exciting aspect of dentistry and by no means should be considered the "final word." We show the business assistant assuming a key position in the management of the dental business office, since this role is now beginning to emerge as vital in dental assistant education.

We wish to emphasize that any fees or data cited in this book are only examples and are not to be perceived as a norm for any geographic area. Furthermore, we know that not all dentists are male and not all dental auxiliaries are female. Please do not construe any personal pronoun in this book as being chauvinistic.

This book has not been completed by our efforts alone. We would like to extend our special thanks to our husbands, Charles Finkbeiner and

James Patt, for their continuous support and patience and to our students, who made it all seem worthwhile.

Special appreciation should be given to Joseph Chasteen, D.D.S., M.S., Robert Klinesteker, D.D.S., Virginia Klinesteker, R.D.H., R.D.A., Robert McPherson, D.D.S., Ruth Menard, C.D.A., Betty Gross, C.D.A., and Shirley Wilson, C.D.A., R.D.A., who represent only a few of our colleagues who have given us encouragement and kept us attuned to the current needs of the profession.

We are most appreciative for the illustrations and materials provided us by Linda Dinsmor, Larry Ulrich of Sycom Co., Madison, Wisconsin; Van Steed of Creative Systems, Southfield, Michigan; Samuel S. Rizzo, Dental Office Computer Systems, Inc., Farmington Hills, Michigan; and Cathy Kiernan of Delta Dental of Michigan. We are grateful, too, for the word processing assistance Phyllis Bostwick gave us in completing this revision.

Betty Ladley Finkbeiner
Jerry Crowe Patt

CONTENTS

1   The Business Assistant in Dentistry

Behavioral Objectives

The business assistant will:
- Identify the duties of the business assistant
- Explain types of productivity
- List hints for success in a job on the dental team

The traditional education of the dentist has placed great emphasis on developing a highly competent diagnostician and clinician but has left a noticeable void in the area of practice management. With TEAM (Training in Auxiliary Management) concepts implemented in dental schools, a greater demand for dental care, expanding group practices, and more concern for public relations in dentistry, a greater emphasis is being placed on business management.

As the modern dentist accepts this new role of dentist/administrator, he accepts the responsibility of delegating expanded intraoral duties to the appropriate clinical assistants, more extraoral duties to the laboratory technician, and additional responsibility to the business assistant.

Who is the Business Assistant?

It is becoming increasingly difficult for dentists to continue to hire inexperienced personnel to manage the business office. In addition to having a broad knowledge of dentistry, the business assistant should be curious, highly organized, be able to accept responsibility, make decisions, have an understanding of business machines, possess skills in management, and be able to communicate with people.

Few data are available, but it seems that in the past dentists have hired persons with secretarial background and little knowledge of dentistry, or high school graduates with minimal experience, or promoted a chairside assistant to the position of business assistant. (This latter arrangement, if the assistant were willing to accept the transition, would seem to have a distinct advantage.) A more desirable approach is to hire a person with education in both business and dental assisting.

Duties of the Business Assistant

Ultimately as the dental team expands, it is likely more management duties will be delegated to the business assistant.

In large, multiple auxiliary dental practices, more than one business assistant will be employed. It is likely that one will be delegated the duties of office manager and the other(s) assigned many of the clerical duties. Duties for which the business assistant may be asked to assume responsibility are listed in the box on p. 2. As you review this list, you will see that the business assistant is a vital link in communication, efficiency, and productivity of the dental office.

COMMON DUTIES OF THE DENTAL OFFICE ASSISTANT

1. Type letters in proper style and with correct spelling and punctuation.
2. Transcribe from shorthand notes or machine.
3. Prepare outgoing mail.
4. Greet patients.
5. Understand patient needs.
6. Use the telephone efficiently.
7. Type addresses on envelopes.
8. Make carbon copies.
9. Open, read, sort, and classify incoming mail.
10. Know when and how to send telegrams and understand the various telegraphic services.
11. Introduce patients and other visitors to the doctor.
12. Use a variety of office machines.
13. Maintain accounting records.
14. Handle bank transactions for the doctor.
15. Make travel reservations and plan trips.
16. Prepare checks.
17. Weigh mail and figure postage.
18. Reconcile a bank statement.
19. Maintain a recall system.
20. Maintain an inventory system.
21. Prepare packages for shipment.
22. Order supplies.
23. Receive supplies and check invoices.
24. Stuff envelopes.
25. Place long distance calls.
26. Proofread.
27. Compose and type letters with or without instructions as to the content.
28. Make appointments for patients.
29. Confirm patient appointments for each day.
30. Prepare laboratory requisitions.
31. Type clinical charts.
32. Know how to use various filing systems.
33. Prepare monthly statements.
34. Understand the use and care of office supplies and automated equipment.
35. Obtain health history from patients.
36. Prepare insurance forms.
37. Use a credit bureau.
38. Use a collection agency.
39. Age accounts and handle delinquent accounts.
40. Prepare consultation materials.
41. Discuss financial arrangements with patients.
42. Organize the business office for efficiency.
43. Have an understanding of all dental procedures to enable you to answer patients' questions.
44. Send greeting cards to patients.
45. Prepare tax forms.
46. Set up budget or bank plans with patients.
47. Design an office manual.
48. Coordinate staff responsibilities.

Human Relations on the Dental Team

Human relations in the dental office often is described as the relationships between the staff and the patient. It is more than that. Others describe the characteristics of good human relations as the ability to be friendly, courteous, and flexible, to get along with others, and practice good manners. It is all of these and yet more.

Human relations is more than getting people to like you. It is knowing how to resolve an unpleasant situation that can arise between you and another person. It is understanding the reasons for another's reactions. It is knowing how to rebuild a deteriorating relationship. It is knowing how to work under pressure and demands made by sometimes unfair supervisors.

Since dentistry is a business, human relations must be understood in terms of productivity. As you join a dental team, you will be expected not only to maintain human relations but also to be able to perform and increase productivity. It is impossible to separate human relations from productivity. One cannot substitute for the other. The doctor will expect you to carry your share of the load. However, getting the work done is only one part of the success story. You must be able to do this work in a manner that is sensitive to those with whom you are working. It must be done in an atmosphere free of antagonism and one in which all members of the dental team can work effectively.

Productivity is important in management. Productivity is not only doing specific duties but also how these duties are performed. The profession of dentistry must be concerned both with productivity and ways of increasing employee morale.

There are two types of productivity on the dental team: individual and group. Each member of the team has a current level of productivity. Although it may vary from day to day, this is the amount of work the individual accomplishes in a given amount of time under specific conditions. Fig. 1-1 illustrates this level of productivity for a business assistant we shall call Debbie, who works in the office of Dr. Lake. The line at the top indicates her current productivity. This is not her maximum or potential level of productivity, which, as with most employees, is greater than her current level of productivity. Fig. 1-2 denotes the potential level of productivity in the shaded area marked by the dotted line. The difference, shown in Fig. 1-3, is the productivity gap. This gap will likely never be closed completely, but it should be as narrow as possible to maintain maximum productivity. This same procedure can be followed for each member of the dental team. Fig. 1-4 shows the production level of each assistant working in Dr. Lake's office. Obviously, as the number of team members increases, the greater the variables will be.

Fig. 1-5 denotes the group productivity when the production level of each assistant is diagramed in a group measurement. Group productivity is not simply the sum of the individuals' productivity. Group productivity will vary according to the ability of the individuals to work together in the group. Note that there is a group productivity gap just as there is an individual productivity gap. A change of any one member of the staff will also change the group productivity and thus the productivity gap.

It is important that the individual dental assistant try to close the gap between current production and potential production. Also, the doctor should attempt to close the gap between the team's current productivity and it's potential. One of the best ways to accomplish this change is to reduce the gap of each individual. The interdependence among members of the dental team cannot be ignored. The way one employee reacts to another is vital in team production. This part of human relations cannot be overlooked and must be resolved within the office to promote greater individual productivity and, as a result, an increased level of productivity for the team.

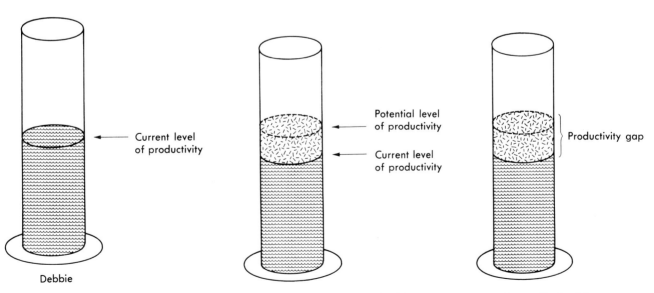

Fig. 1-1. Current productivity.   **Fig. 1-2.** Potential productivity.   **Fig. 1-3.** Productivity gap.

Fig. 1-4. Productivity levels for each member of dental team.

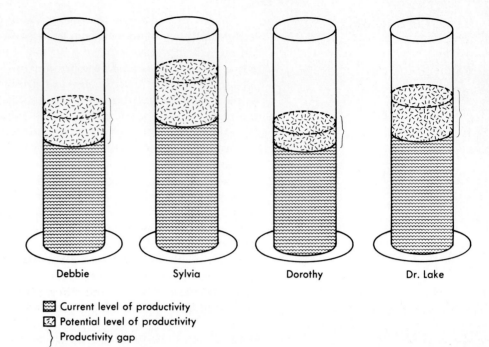

Debbie   Sylvia   Dorothy   Dr. Lake

▨ Current level of productivity
▧ Potential level of productivity
} Productivity gap

Fig. 1-5. Group productivity.

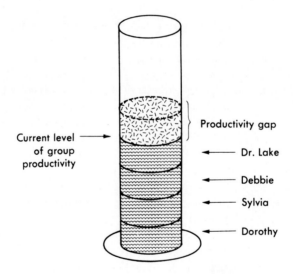

Productivity gap

Current level
of group →
productivity

← Dr. Lake
← Debbie
← Sylvia
← Dorothy

Hints for Success as Part of the Dental Team

When beginning a new job on the dental health team, you should gear yourself to success. The following suggestions can help.

Learning the Names of Members of the Staff. Learning and remembering names of your immediate associates should not be difficult. If the staff is large, learning names of persons not in your immediate department may be more difficult. It is wise to learn the names as quickly as possible. It may even be wise to maintain a list of names and the position of each employee until you are able to remember them.

Establishing Social Friendships. Most offices do not object if employees develop personal friendships with other employees. However, many traps can develop on your first days on a new job. One of these is developing a close relationship with one or two people which will cost you friendship with others at a later time. Office cliques frequently create rivalry. Although you must possess a friendly attitude toward other employees in the office, you need not feel you must participate in all the social activities or interests the others have. You should, however, avoid a superior attitude that can be interpreted as "snobbish."

Using a Notebook and Calendar. When you begin your new job, many unfamiliar rules, regulations, and information will be given to you. To avoid misunderstanding or neglecting important information, develop the "notebook habit" and write down each bit of information. It is surprising how many successful people use this system.

Observing Office Hours. In most instances the office hours have been determined prior to your arrival. The efficiency of an office depends on your being prompt at all times. Your tardiness will only delay the work process for which you are responsible. You should protect your means of transportation at all times. It is your responsibility to anticipate inclement weather and compensate for any potential delay. *It is better to be twenty minutes early than two minutes late.* The doctor will not be interested in your excuses.

Using Judgment in Working Overtime and Taking Breaks. Employees sometimes try to impress the employer by working extra hours or skipping lunch hours or breaks. However, you should avoid continual overtime and loss of lunch hours because it may cause friction with other employees. Your actions may be misinterpreted and other employees may make life miserable for you. This does not mean you cannot use your discretion on those days when legitimate emergencies arise and your presence is necessary in maintaining office efficiency.

Not Flaunting Your Education and Abilities. Nothing is more irritating than for a new employee to constantly inform other employees about his or her exceptional abilities. It is better to prove your ability through your work than to tell everyone about your great potential. Your coworkers may have had many years of experience and you might learn something from them if you give them a chance to help you.

Maintaining Office Policies. Most offices have established policies for grooming and uniform styles. You should carefully review the office policy and adhere to it. In addition, you should take home any other handbooks the office uses for its employees and read them carefully so that you will be well informed. Should you not understand any portion, it is wise to ask for clarification to avoid making an embarrassing mistake.

Being Yourself. As you make your first impression in the office, it is wise to be yourself. Remember, you may admire characteristics in another person, but you cannot be that person. If you attempt to be someone else, you only destroy yourself and all of the finer parts of your character. Be yourself and you will be a happier person.

Asking for a Raise

When you begin work, pay increments may be discussed and you will be aware that raises are given after six months or a year of successful employment. However, if pay increments have not been discussed and you have completed a year of employment, when and how can the subject be discussed?

Before approaching the doctor about a raise, several factors should be considered. A salary discussion should provide a two-way communication that will solve the problem.

1. Have you performed your duties well enough to deserve a raise?
2. Have you improved or advanced your assisting skills since beginning the job?
3. Have you been cooperative with other members of the dental team?
4. Has the doctor's productivity increased because of your assistance?
5. Do economic factors within the practice, as well as the economy, warrant a raise?

After serious thought has been given to the factors mentioned above, and you feel that you deserve a raise, how will you approach the doctor? Select a time when the work schedule permits enough time to discuss the subject. Do not wait until the end of the day when the doctor is tired and ready to leave the office. It is also not wise to start the day by asking for a raise, especially if the schedule is rather heavy.

Let the doctor know why you feel you deserve a raise. If he asks why you need one, be prepared to answer; for example, the cost of living is rising, transportation costs, insurance, or some unexpected expense.

Very often, employees do not assert themselves enough to make the doctor aware that a raise should be given. If you become passive and content with a salary, naturally you will continue to be paid at this rate; however, if your professional skills are an asset, and because of these skills the doctor can perform his job to greater efficiency, then a raise should be given.

If the employer cannot raise your salary, here are a few alternatives to a salary increase:

1. Uniform allowance (for example, the cost of five uniforms per year)
2. Retirement plan
3. Health insurance
4. Dental care (for self or family or both)
5. Holiday bonus
6. Profit sharing plan (a plan which might provide the assistant with 2% of the accounts receivable, plus receipts)
7. Travel and expense to professional meetings
8. Dues to professional organizations

If you have been unsuccessful in getting a raise, express your appreciation for the doctor's understanding and consideration and consider your alternatives; of course, if you receive a raise, be sure to thank the responsible person.

Salary matters should be treated confidentially and are not matters to be discussed with other members of the team. Salary problems destroy positive attitudes and productivity and should be resolved as quickly as possible.

Job Termination

Terminating a job can be an obstacle for some individuals, especially when the change of jobs is from one private practice to another within the same general locale. When changing jobs, be sure the change is to your advantage. Circumstances over which you have no control may be the reason for a change in jobs. Whatever the reason for terminating the job, do it ethically:

1. Give the reason for leaving the job.
2. Give sufficient notice, at least two weeks or a longer time if your job requires an extensive training period for a new assistant.
3. Write a letter of resignation as a follow-up of your verbal resignation.
4. Do not discuss the termination of your job with other members of the team until you are ready to inform the doctor that you will be leaving. The grapevine is a poor method of informing.
5. Good ethics require that if you have terminated a job where there have been serious conflicts, it is best to leave these conflicts where they originated and not carry these feelings to another job. When beginning a new position, you should not make negative comments about a former employer.

Exercises

1. List twenty-five common duties of the business assistant.
2. Explain why human relations are important in interpersonal relationships.
3. Explain the difference between individual productivity and group productivity. What is meant by the productivity gap?
4. Discuss six suggestions for success on the job.
5. Discuss the procedure for:
   a. Asking for a raise
   b. Terminating a job.

Suggested Activities

On p. 287 are suggested activities that relate to this chapter.

Bibliography

Chapman, E.N.: Your attitude is showing—a primer on human relations, ed. 2, Palo Alto, CA, 1972, Science Research Associates, Inc.

Department of Health, Education & Welfare, Public Health Service, Health Resources Administration, Bureau of Health Resources Development, Division of Dentistry: Guidelines for the dental TEAM program, Bethesda, MD, April, 1975 (revised).

Fulton, P.J.: General office procedures for colleges, ed. 8, Cincinnati, 1983, South-Western Publishing Co.

2   Applying for a Position in the Dental Profession

Behavioral Objectives

The business assistant will:
- Make explicit a philosophy for dental assisting
- Write an effective letter of application with a resume
- Prepare for a job interview
- Make an appropriate follow-up to an interview
- Identify personality and hygiene characteristics that need improvement

Philosophy

Before seeking employment, you should determine your needs and make explicit your life goals and the philosophy that is consistent with them. Unfortunately, a dental assistant may accept the first job offer with little consideration given to how her philosophy coincides with the philosophy of her prospective employer. Carefully evaluate yourself and establish some realistic goals. Then ask yourself, the following questions: Are my professional, moral, and social values compatible with those of my prospective employer? In what type of working environment do I wish to be associated, a solo practice or a large group practice? Which of my skills in dental assisting do I wish to use to the greatest extent? What are my strengths? What are my weaknesses? How can I compensate for my weaknesses? What do I want to be doing in five years; in ten years? How important are salary, hours, and location?

Once you have written your philosophy toward life and enumerated your goals, don't forget that these goals will be ever changing, and you undoubtedly will reevaluate your philosophy as you gain confidence from your new experiences.

Potential Areas of Employment

Private Practice. The dental assistant may seek employment in a private practitioner's office or a group practice or clinic comprised of several dentists. A dental practice may be general, in which all phases of dental treatment are rendered for a patient, or it may be limited to one of the specialties of dentistry recognized by the American Dental Association; these are endodontics, orthodontics, oral surgery, oral pathology, pedodontics, periodontics, prosthodontics, and public health. In private practice, the dental assistant may find a position limited specifically to chairside assisting, office management, laboratory duties, or a combination of all these responsibilities. Private practice affords many opportunities to work closely with the doctor and patients, diversification of duties, individuality, and a great number of personal responsibilities. With increased value placed on the highly skilled dental assistant, compensation and benefits will continue to increase.

Institutional Dentistry. With increased interest of federal, state, and local governments in dental care delivery, an even greater number of facilities are being established to provide more dental services for the public. One institution that should be considered as a source of employment is the dental school. Schools offer many areas of potential employment, from working with undergraduates at chairside to teaching in auxiliary utilization programs. Other institutions are a part of the Civil Service programs and offer employment in prisons, public clinics, and Veteran's Administration Hospitals. Additionally, hospitals, some of which are associated closely with dental schools, offer employment in their surgery departments. The dental assistant working in an institution has the opportunity to work with a larger staff than is possible in private dental practice, diversification of duties, participation in newly developed techniques, potential advancement to several levels of supervision, and possibly more liberal vacations (in learning institutions vacations are often coordinated with school calendars).

Insurance Offices. This phase of employment is especially appealing to the dental assistant who aspires to perform secretarial duties and become involved in management. With the advent of dental insurance coverage, more companies are seeking highly qualified dental assistants to work in management positions, since a broad knowledge of dentistry is an asset to their business. A position in insurance may also involve public-speaking activities and travel.

Research. Hospitals and dental schools hire many dental assistants to work in research laboratories. Persons who enjoy working with mathematical computations and details and who enjoy being independent often seek positions in research.

Dental Manufacturers. One area of potential employment that should not be overlooked is the dental manufacturers who employ dental assistants for sales and teaching. Such employment would limit contact with dentistry to one specific area of products but would offer a great opportunity to travel throughout the country and meet people.

Teaching. Numerous colleges and universities have developed occupational education programs that include dental assisting. A graduate of a dental assistant program who is a Certified Dental Assistant (CDA) or Registered Dental Assistant (RDA) may transfer into a baccalaureate degree program. Anyone who has broad experience in dental assisting, is highly motivated to teach, and is patient and objective should perhaps contact a college or university about entrance into their program. Another source of information is the American Dental Assistants' Association.

Where Do You Begin to Find Employment Opportunities?

After surveying some of these potential areas of employment, where do you begin looking for the right job? Many prospects are available, and several different avenues may be used.

School Placement. The school placement office or faculty instructors are often notified of job opportunities in the area. Instructors often know employers who are interested in hiring new graduates, and they also know their students' qualifications and abilities. Schools often spend a great deal of time obtaining information regarding potential job opportunities and take a great deal of pride in placing their graduates.

Newspaper Advertisements. Both local and out-of-area newspapers provide classified sections of jobs available. Advertisements appearing in the classified section will state the qualifications needed for the job and other details relating to the job (Fig. 2-1). However, in some instances, the employer will not give the name of the practice or telephone number, but will place a "blind ad" asking the applicant to submit a resume (Fig. 2-2). This type of ad should not be overlooked, because it becomes the employer's first means of screening applicants. Remember that while first impressions are not necessarily the most accurate, they often are the most influential. A little more initiative is necessary on the applicant's part when she must construct a resume rather than pick up the telephone and call for an interview. The prospective employer will use the letter of application and resume to evaluate the applicant's typing skills, communication skills, and neatness.

Employment Agencies. There are free employment agencies available as well as private employment agencies. Most states provide an employment service and applicants may register with them without charge.

Private employment agencies, which are service enterprises, provide many good job opportunities, but not without charge. Before registering with an employment agency, it is wise to determine the reputation of the agency. This can be done locally or through the National Employment Association in Washington, D.C. After selecting a reputable agency, the applicant should determine testing and placement procedures.

Other sources for job opportunities not to be overlooked are friends, relatives, business associates, local dental assistant societies, dental associations, dental supply houses, and dental schools. If a friend is leaving a particular job and knows you are interested in this particular area of dentistry and available for work, a good recommendation is always welcome.

Letter of Application

When applying for available jobs, the applicant must write a letter of application and submit a personal data sheet or resume.

Let's begin with the letter of application, a letter which may very well be the most important business letter you ever write. The prime objective of the letter of application is to make your reader interested in your skills and abilities and grant you an interview. How can this best be accomplished?

First, the letter must be attractive. It will be typed in correct form, with correct spelling and grammar and typed on acceptable stationery, preferably buff or white bond paper.

Although the letter of application is written stating your qualifications, etc., each sentence should not begin with "I." You can best accomplish this by putting the employer's needs first and stressing what you have to offer as a potential employee and how your skills will benefit the employer.

The first paragraph should state the objective for writing the letter. You are applying for a particular job which was advertised, or you have been informed of the job through another source.

The second paragraph lets the reader learn a little about you and why you are qualified for the job. You should always make positive and accurate statements about your ability. You should provide facts that accurately describe what the employer can expect from you as an employee. You want to convince a prospective employer that you (1) know what the job entails, (2) are able to do the job, (3) can get along with others, (4) are dependable, and (5) are able to fit the dental office image. Detailed infor-

Fig. 2-1. Newspaper advertisement.

Certified Dental Assistant who is ambitious
and experienced in four-handed dentistry.
Duties include chairside, laboratory, and
business office management in a general
practice. Inquire: Joseph W. Lake, D.D.S.,
611 Main St. S.E.. Grand Rapids. MI 49502

Fig. 2-2. Blind ad.

Dental Office Manager: Interested in a
challenging position? A group dental practice
is looking for an office manager. You must be
ambitious, be able to supervise auxiliary staff,
work effectively under pressure, use good
judgment and be able to accept responsibility.
Reply: Box #2589, Grand Rapids News,
Grand Rapids, MI 49502

Fig. 2-3. Letter of application.

                                           5281 Kalamazoo Ave., S.E.
                                           Grand Rapids, MI 49507
                                           June 15, 19--

Joseph W. Lake, D.D.S.
611 Main Street S.E.
Grand Rapids, MI 49502

Dear Dr. Lake:

     Your advertisement of June 12, 19-- in the Grand Rapids News prompted
me to write this letter. You asked for a dental assistant who is educated
in four-handed dentistry, gets along with people, and possesses management
skills. May I be considered as an applicant for this job?

     During the past year and a half, I have taken courses at Kent Community
College, Grand Rapids, Michigan to prepare me as a certified dental assistant.
You will see from the enclosed resume that I have successfully completed
courses in dental assisting that will be valuable to your practice. I have
had considerable clinical and business office experience.

     May I have an interview at your convenience? You may contact me at
111-2817 after 3:00 p.m. any day of the week.

                                   Sincerely,

                                   Deborah L. Benson, C.D.A.

Enclosure

mation regarding your course work and related job experience is best outlined on your resume.

Your third paragraph should ask for an interview and make it convenient for the reader to respond. For example, indicate how you can be reached by telephone at a certain time.

See Fig. 2-3 to see how Deborah Benson wrote her letter of application when applying for a dental assistant position in the office of Joseph W. Lake, D.D.S.

If you have been informed of a job opening by an instructor or friend, perhaps there isn't sufficient time to write a letter of application, and a telephone call is required. What procedure is best in this situation? First, indicate to the individual receiving your call who you are and why you are calling. Second, explain how you learned about the position. Finally, if the job is available, ask for an interview. Before going for the interview, prepare a resume to take with you.

Resume

The resume, personal data sheet, or personal history should be prepared to accompany the letter of application. Remember, your objective is to be granted an interview; therefore, you want to impress your reader with a resume that is concise and a positive presentation of your abilities and qualifications.

When preparing the resume make several copies. For example, you should have one for yourself when going for an interview. Even though several copies of the data sheet will be needed, each one should be individually typed or printed by a commercial printer. A carbon copy should not be sent to an employer but may be used for your personal files.

The information on the resume should be arranged so that it presents your qualifications and abilities to the greatest advantage. A typical arrangement is shown in the following:

Personal Data. Personal data include:
1. Full name
2. Address
3. Telephone number
4. Social Security number
5. Health (optional)

Objective. A positive statement concerning the sort of position you seek should be included in the resume.

Education. Include relevant information regarding your educational background. List all colleges and universities attended and the date you graduated. (List most recent schools first.) List diplomas or degrees, as well as awards and scholarships or special achievements. Courses that you took when completing the dental assistant program might be listed (for example, dental science, dental laboratory procedures, clinical practice, dental roentgenology, and dental practice management).

Work Experience. Begin with your last job and include dates of employment, name and address of employer, position held, and a brief description of the job. Summer and part-time jobs may be lumped in a single category; however, if work experiences have been limited, you may wish to list them separately.

In some instances, if your work experience is more recent than your education, the work experience should be listed before your education. At this point in your career, work experience is of greater value to a prospective employer than the education.

Activities. If you have participated in school or community activities, and this information would be valuable to the prospective employer, it should be included. Activities and hobbies often indicate that you are a well-rounded individual and get along well with others.

Fig. 2-4. Resume.

RESUME

PERSONAL DATA

Name: Deborah L. Benson

Address: 5281 Kalamazoo Ave., S. E.
              Grand Rapids, MI 49507

Telephone No: AC 616 - III-2817   Soc. Sec. No: 369-38-5043

Objective: To obtain a job that will utilize my dental assisting skills to a maximum
            in the practice of team dentistry.

EDUCATION

Kent Community College, Grand Rapids, Michigan
Graduated, June 19--, Associate Degree in Dental Assisting, 3.42 Grade Point Average
CDA - May 28, 19--
Related Courses: Dental Science   Clinical Practice
                  Dental Laboratory Procedures   Dental Roentgenology
                  Dental Practice Management
Member of: Kent County Dental Ass't. Assoc., Michigan Dental Ass't. Assoc. and
            American Dental Ass't. Assoc.

South High School, Grand Rapids, Michigan
Graduated, June 19--, College Preparatory

WORK EXPERIENCE

Clinical Practice: January - June, 19--
Xavier University, School of Dentistry
      DAU, Pedodontic, and Crown and Bridge Clinics
Charles Allan, D.D.S. 123 Huron River Drive, S.E. Grand Rapids, Michigan
James Richardson, D.D.S. 2608 Patricia, Wyoming, Michigan
Charles Van Beek, D.D.S. 2426 Naubinway, Franklin, Michigan

Summer Job: June - September, 19--
J. D. Jenks, D.D.S. 1334 Main S. E., Grand Rapids, Michigan

REFERENCES

Ms. Virginia Klinesteker, Instructor   Ms. Dorothy Van Dyke, Owner
Kent Community College   Princess Dress Shoppe
Grand Rapids, Michigan 49502   6341 Division East
Business Telephone: AC 616 - 111-6300   Grand Rapids, MI 49506
Home Telephone: AC 616 - 111-1162   Business Telephone: AC 616 - 111-7210
                                         Home Telephone: AC 616 - 111-7622

Charles Allan, D.D.S.
123 Huron River Drive, S.E.
Grand Rapids, Michigan 49506
Business Telephone: AC 616 - 111-7108
Home Telephone: AC 616 - 111-1212

References. List at least two people who can vouch for your abilities and skills and one character reference. If your work experience has been limited, list instructors or laboratory supervisors who can evaluate your abilities. Always obtain the individual's permission to use his or her name as a reference and be sure that person is willing to give you a good recommendation. The person's full name and address, title (if any), and telephone numbers should be listed. You may not wish to list your references. If so, indicate they are available upon request.

Remember, do not give information on the resume that might be detrimental to you. Details can be given when you are interviewed. At the interview be prepared to discuss your weaknesses honestly, confidently, and in a way that puts your present self in the best light.

See Fig. 2-4 to see how Deborah Benson prepared her resume to accompany her letter of application.

Filling Out the Application Form

The type of dental assisting job for which you are applying will determine the detail and complexity of the application form. You may have had the opportunity to complete the application form before arriving for the interview or you may be asked to complete the form when you arrive. See Fig. 2-5 for an example of an application used for private practice.

Regardless of the job for which you are applying, there are several things to keep in mind when completing the form. If possible, try to obtain two forms-one to use as a working copy, the other to submit to the employer.

Before filling out the application form read through the application very thoroughly and avoid asking unnecessary questions. The application form is often used as the first employment test. It tests your ability to follow directions, as well as neatness.

The directions may indicate that the form can be typed or written. If you are required to complete the form in your own handwriting, this may be another test of neatness and also give the employer a sample of how well or poorly you write.

Be sure to answer all questions. If the question does not relate to you, write N/A (not applicable) or draw a line through the question. The employer then realizes you have read the question and not overlooked it.

Be truthful when answering the questions. Dates, names, and places need to be accurate. Make a list of your former addresses, schools, and even your grandparents' names to take along when going for the interview. Occasionally some forms ask for detailed and specific family background information. It is better to have the information available even if it is not needed. Be sure that no discrepancies exist between your date of birth and your age. If you are residing at a temporary address, be sure to give a permanent address. Be particularly careful with your spelling. A small pocket dictionary is a great item to take along as a handy reference.

Preparing for the Personal Interview

The day you receive a call or letter from a prospective employer, you will be elated and pleased to know that someone is interested in your qualifications after reading them on the resume and now wishes to meet you in person. This elation is immediately followed by a feeling of fear—fear of the unknown. You may or may not know anything about this prospective position, but one thing is certain, you do know yourself by this time. Let us take a look at Deborah Benson as she prepares herself for an interview with Dr. Lake. At a later time, you should go through each of these steps and apply them to your situation.

Fig. 2-5. Application for employment. (Courtesy Sycom.)

EMPLOYMENT APPLICATION

All information listed on this application will be considered and handled as personal and confidential. Please write or print legibly.

Date _____

NAME _____ PHONE NO. _____

MAILING ADDRESS _____ SS# _____
No.   Street   City   State   Zip

How long have you lived in this area? _____ Are you over 18 yrs. of age and under 70? Yes _____ No _____

Are you known by Schools / References by another name? Yes _____ No _____ If yes by what name? _____

Position interested in: _____ If offered employment when can you start _____
(Date)

Will transportation to work be a problem for you? Yes _____ No _____

Can your vacation be arranged most any time? Yes _____ No _____ If no, when? _____

Is there any reason why you could not be bonded? Yes _____ No _____ Do you wish employment: Full time _____

Part time _____ Hours per week _____

Does the sight of blood bother you? Yes _____ No _____

Number of days missed from work/school in last year because of illness or injury: _____

List any physical defects or chronic diseases you think may interfere with your ability to perform the job you are presently applying for:

_____
_____
_____

EDUCATION

	Elementary	High	College/University	Professional
School Name				
Years Completed: (Circle)	4 5 6 7 8	9 10 11 12	1 2 3 4	1 2 3 4
Diploma/Degree				
Describe Course Of Study:				
Describe Specialized Training, Apprenticeship, Skills, Seminars, Courses, Extra-Curricular Activities				

SKILLS:

	(circle)			(circle)	
Typing (Speed _____)	Yes	No	Pour Models	Yes	No
Shorthand (Speed _____)	Yes	No	Cavitron	Yes	No
Bookkeeping - Pegboard	Yes	No	Cast Inlays	Yes	No
Dictation Equipment	Yes	No	Plaque Control Instruction	Yes	No
Handling Group Insurance	Yes	No	Oral Evacuator	Yes	No
Take X-Rays	Yes	No	Knowledge of Dental Instruments	Yes	No
Panoramic X-Rays	Yes	No	Knowledge of Dental Terms	Yes	No
Other: (Describe if yes)	Yes	No	Data Processing	Yes	No

_____
_____
_____

This employer provides equal opportunity to all persons without regard to handicap, race, color, religion, sex, age or national origin.

Form 113 1980 SYCOM, Madison, WI Printed in U.S.A.   Over

Continued.

Fig. 2-5, cont'd. Application for employment.

EMPLOYMENT RECORD · List most recent employer first:

Name of Employer		
Address		
Supervisor & Telephone Number		
Title & Description of your job		
Dates of Employment	Start	Last
Earnings	Start	Last
Reason for leaving		

Name of Employer		
Address		
Supervisor & Telephone Number		
Title & Description of your job		
Dates of Employment	Start	Last
Earnings	Start	Last
Reason for leaving		

Name of Employer		
Address		
Supervisor & Telephone Number		
Title & Description of your job		
Dates of Employment	Start	Last
Earnings	Start	Last
Reason for leaving		

REFERENCES (not former employers or relatives):

NAME	ADDRESS	TYPE BUSINESS

In the course of making an employment decision, this employer makes it a practice to verify with previous employers information such as dates of employment, description of job duties, attendance records, reason for leaving, etc. If there are any employers you wish we not contact, please indicate their names below and reasons why:

_____

I understand that if I am employed and any statement herein is not true, I may be released immediately, I will be paid only through the day of release and this employer may cancel any rights to accrued benefits.

_____   _____
Date   Signature

What Do I Wear? Deborah has decided to wear something that looks businesslike. She has a new outfit that she would like to have worn but could not decide if it was the proper thing to wear. (Remember, if you question whether an outfit is right or not, don't wear it.) Debbie has washed her hair, and styled it in a style in which she feels comfortable and one that looks good on her. She wears a moderate amount of makeup and avoids too heavy a fragrance of cologne. Debbie knows that her personal appearance is an important part of the interview and has followed the old adage "first appearances are lasting ones." You may know all the answers and possess a lot of skill, but you must win the approval of the doctor before you will ever have an opportunity to display these skills.

What Do I Take With Me? The day Deborah received the call for the interview she wrote down the time, place, and name of the interviewer. She also decided what she should take with her to the interview. She has prepared her materials which include a ballpoint pen, a pencil, an eraser, a small spiral notebook, and a pocket dictionary. In addition, she has obtained a copy of her grades in case Dr. Lake wishes to have this record for his evaluation. Debbie has also included a copy of her resume in case she needs to make reference to it. In her notebook, Debbie has listed many of her outstanding characteristics which she may wish to bring to the attention of Dr. Lake. Also, she has a list of questions that she hopes he will cover during the interview and if not, she may ask him about some of her concerns.

The Personal Interview

Deborah arrives early at Dr. Lake's office where her first contact is with the office manager. The office manager plays an important role in Dr. Lake's office so it is important to be friendly to her. Deborah is cordial to her and says, "Good morning, I am Deborah Benson, and I have a 10:30 appointment for an interview with Dr. Lake." The office manager acknowledges her and asks her to complete an application form similar to that shown in Fig. 2-5. After the form is completed, the office manager will escort her in to meet Dr. Lake. If she does not introduce Debbie, Debbie is ready to say, "Good morning, Dr. Lake, I am Deborah Benson." Dr. Lake asks Debbie to be seated and Debbie is prepared to begin answering his questions as she looks directly at him. Debbie knows that she must speak clearly and avoid being evasive. An evasive answer will leave a doubt in the interviewer's mind.

In general, the applicant should be responsive and answer in complete sentences. Refer to the following boxed material on characteristics to avoid during an interview.

THINGS TO AVOID DURING THE INTERVIEW

1. Being too aggressive
2. Talking about salary and hours immediately
3. Chewing gum
4. Lacking enthusiasm
5. Lacking a neat appearance
6. Using little or no eye contact
7. Appearing preoccupied
8. Using poor grammar
9. Being vague
10. Wearing too much makeup
11. Lacking curiosity

The following questions are ones which Deborah encountered during her interview and are common ones you should be prepared to answer.

What Are Your Long-range and Short-range Goals? This is a good question to begin with since it opens the door for you to talk about yourself. When you established your philosophy, you gave attention to your goals and now is the time to explain them verbally. Don't feel the interviewer is being too personal since this is one of the greatest methods of finding out about an applicants' plans and interests. Be sincere and honest, but brief and concise.

How Would You Describe Yourself? This brief description should say more than "I like to work with people." It should include two or three of your strongest personal characteristics. Debbie described herself to Dr. Lake as being a person who "enjoys getting up each morning and spending some time outside with her animals where, in the quiet, she could organize her thoughts and work for the day." She also told Dr. Lake she enjoyed being around people who had a good sense of humor and has found out she often laughs at herself, a good way to accept criticism.

What Do You Consider Your Greatest Weakness? Each person has areas of weaknesses, some of which are a result of inexperience while others perhaps are limitations to one's ability. Debbie was honest with Dr. Lake when she told him "I don't enjoy laboratory work, but perhaps that is because my experience has been limited. In school we had a great deal of clinical experience at chairside, but I have not had as much experience in the laboratory area. If you would like to have me perform extensive duties in this area, I would be most willing to work outside of my regular hours to increase my skills." She went on further to state that, "Until I began my college program, I was always turned off by people nagging me and became disinterested in them, but now from my experience at school I have found that if I organize myself and complete my work on time, I have no reason for people to nag me. Further, I am very proud of my work when I complete it."

Why Should I Hire You? This is a difficult question to answer, since you may not really know the needs of this office. If, however, you have previously determined what the position will involve, you should be able to emphasize your strengths in these areas. For instance, Dr. Lake was interested in hiring a person at chairside who would be able to work in the business office in six months when his office manager would be on maternity leave. Deborah explained to him that she felt her broad clinical experience had provided her with enough background to work well at chairside. She knew all the basic operative set-ups and needed only learn his special techniques as they applied to any given procedure. Further, during her experiences she had worked with numerous people and she adapted well to new people and environments. She went on to explain that she felt within six months she could have a good working knowledge of Dr. Lake's office and would be well prepared to take over in the business office during his assistant's absence. She also enumerated to Dr. Lake the various skills she had obtained in the business management area.

You should avoid bragging, but be honest and discuss an application of your skills to the given situation.

Will You Be Willing to Work for $— a Week? Unfortunately, private practitioners do not have a well-defined salary scale and system of benefits. This situation is improving, and many dentists are beginning to follow the system of institutions that do have a well-defined salary scale. In Chapter 3, specific benefits are described in the discussion concerning management and decision-making. The salary is often discussed without the assistant raising the question. If the salary the doctor offers you is lower than you are willing to accept, you may reply that you had hoped to start at a higher salary, but that you are willing to have an opportunity to display your ability and value to him. This will undoubtedly result in further discussion, whereupon you should be prepared to give firm answers on what you will accept. Also, you should inquire if there are benefits that might offset the lower salary. Deborah was offered a lower salary and replied, "I feel I have the skills you need and it is going to save you a great deal of time in not having to teach me about all the technical skills. I would be willing to start at the lower salary if you will explain to me what the total salary scale is and how I will be evaluated for salary raises. I would like the opportunity to advance by merit or production since I am certain you will be pleased with my ability and production in your office." Dr. Lake explained the numerous benefits and outlined the salary system to Deborah. Remember, salary is not the primary aspect of the job, but you must be able to earn enough to support yourself and not eliminate some of the more enjoyable things in life. Also, the benefits of a job often outweigh the basic salary, so don't overlook this aspect.

To avoid friction that might arise at a later date, you should feel free to discuss salary and benefits. You should enter the interview well prepared to discuss benefits such as profit sharing, health insurance, uniform allowances, retirement plans, education allowances, leaves, and vacations.

Ending the Interview

An interview is not a lengthy process and is often terminated with a tour of the office. Do not be overflattering to the staff, but thank them for their time before you leave. You may not receive a job offer during the interview, since the doctor may have other applicants to interview. However, you may inquire as to when he anticipates arriving at a decision. Remember, do not be discouraged if you do not get the job. Each interview is a learning experience and should not be treated as a disappointment.

Following Up the Interview

A good follow-up letter (Fig. 2-6) should be written two or three days following the interview. This is an indication to the interviewer that you are interested in the position, and it may place you as a priority applicant for the position.

The follow-up letter does not have to be long. It simply restates your interest in the job and mentions some of the facts that interested you about the job.

Another type of follow-up letter may be necessary if you have not had a reply from the prospective employer. If the job is still available and you are interested, it is permissible to call the interviewer in a day or two after the interview. A telephone call lets the interviewer know of your continued interest, but at the same time too many telephone calls can be annoying.

If you decide later that you are not interested in the position, a letter should be written indicating your decision and explaining your decision. Not only is this thoughtful, but also there may be a time when you will find yourself in a position to go back to this employer.

Fig. 2-6. Follow-up letter.

5281 Kalamazoo Ave., S. E.
Grand Rapids, MI 49507
June 25, 19—

Joseph W. Lake, D.D.S.
611 Main Street S. E.
Grand Rapids, MI 49502

Dear Dr. Lake:

Thank you for the interview you gave me yesterday afternoon.

It was my privilege to see such a well-organized dental team. Because of my training, I am confident that I can become an efficient dental assistant and an asset to your dental team.

After you have had a chance to review my application, you will see that I have had considerable work experience.

I am available for work immediately. You may contact me any day of the week by calling 111-2817 after 3:00 p.m.

Sincerely,

Deborah L. Benson, C. D.A.

Self-Evaluation

Regular self-evaluation will be necessary in order to retain your position in the dental office. People often carefully evaluate themselves prior to employment but may become careless after working in the office for a period of time.

Don't become negligent in the evaluation of yourself. As a dental assistant you are constantly in the public eye and must retain a good image in your employer's office. In Figs. 2-7 and 2-8, you will find a checklist of personal and hygienic characteristics that should be referred to regularly.

Additionally, once you have obtained the position you will be required to maintain your skills and obtain new skills as changes take place in dentistry through expanded auxiliary utilization. You should promptly join your professional organizations that provide you with opportunities to learn of educational activities that will provide you with relevant techniques as they become available.

Fig. 2-7. Personal checklist.

Self evaluation
Personal characteristics

The following questions are designed for you to use in evaluation of your own personal characteristics. If you cannot honestly answer a question "yes," then you should spend time in self-improvement in these areas during the coming weeks. REMEMBER—be honest with yourself; you are the person who will benefit the most from such an evaluation.

Self-confidence	Yes	No	Sometimes
1. Do you communicate easily with people?			
2. Are you willing to continue with a job even though you are criticized?			
3. When you have made a decision, do you support your decision?			
4. Do you refrain from bragging?			
5. Do you accept new responsibilities easily?			
Tactfulness			
6. Do you think about what you say before saying it?			
7. Do you practice self-control?			
8. Do you avoid unnecessary interruptions of others' privacy?			
9. Do you make patients feel important?			
10. Are you patient with others?			
11. Do you have empathy for other people?			
Dependability			
12. Are you always on time for work, school, and/or appointments?			
13. Do you pay attention to the details of your work?			
14. Do you avoid being absent except for serious illness?			
15. Do you follow through with your commitments?			
16. Do you stay with a job until it is finished?			
17. Do you always do the job assigned to you?			
Initiative			
18. Do you look for work that needs to be done?			
19. Do you organize your time?			
20. Are you proud of your completed work?			
21. Are you eager to please other people?			
22. Do you accomplish more work than is assigned to you?			
Judgment and decision making			
23. Are you eager to learn new things?			
24. Are you curious about the unknown?			
25. Do you examine all possibilities before making a decision?			
26. Do you evaluate the results of an action before taking it?			
27. Are you interested in continuing education?			
Integrity			
28. Do you respect other people and their property?			
29. Do you avoid discussing confidential information?			
30. Do you refrain from gossip?			
31. Can you be trusted with money that belongs to the office?			
32. Do you tell the truth even though you may suffer the consequences?			

Continued.

Fig. 2-7, cont'd. Personal checklist.

Human relations	Yes	No	Sometimes
33. Do you have a sense of humor?			
34. Are you a good listener?			
35. Do you maintain eye contact when talking to another person?			
36. Can you accept criticism?			
37. Do you avoid being overbearing?			
38. Do you speak first when meeting someone new?			
39. Do you think of others before yourself?			
40. Do you use a person's name when talking to him?			
41. Do you avoid frowning and smile naturally?			

Fig. 2-8. Hygienic checklist.

Self evaluation
Hygiene and grooming characteristics

The following questions are designed for you to use in evaluating your personal hygiene. If you cannot honestly answer a question "yes," then you should spend time in developing a daily routine that will improve your grooming and hygiene habits. REMEMBER—as a member of a health profession you must set a good example of optimum health.

Body hygiene	Yes	No	Sometimes
1. Do you bathe daily?			
2. Do you use a deodorant daily?			
Oral hygiene			
3. Do you brush your teeth at least twice daily?			
4. Do you have regular oral prophylaxis?			
5. Do you have your mouth restored to maximum dental health?			
6. Do you use floss to aid in destruction of plaque?			
Hair			
7. Do you shampoo your hair regularly?			
8. Is your hair always neatly combed?			
9. Is your hair styled to keep it off your face and out of the field of operation?			
10. Is your scalp free of dandruff?			
Hands			
11. Are your nails short, clean, and well manicured?			
12. Do you avoid the use of nail polish?			
13. Are your hands smooth and always clean?			
Eyes			
14. Do you have regular eye examinations?			
15. Are your eyebrows well groomed?			
16. If you wear glasses, are they well fitted and clean?			
17. Do you avoid excessive eye makeup?			
Face			
18. Do you avoid excessive use of makeup?			
19. Is your face clean and free of disease?			
20. Is your face free of dry, scaly areas?			

Fig. 2-8, cont'd. Hygienic checklist.

	Yes	No	Sometimes
General health			
21. Do you get adequate sleep at night?			
22. Do you have an annual physical examination?			
23. Do you exercise daily?			
24. Do you participate in some form of recreation weekly?			
Posture			
25. Do you stand erect?			
26. Do you sit straight in a chair?			
27. Do you wear shoes that are comfortable and proper fitting?			
28. Are your feet free of disease?			
Uniform			
29. Do you wear a clean, wrinkle-free uniform daily?			
30. Are your shoes clean and highly polished?			
31. Is your uniform free of stains and repairs?			
32. Do you wear fresh underwear daily?			
33. Do you avoid excessive use of jewelry?			

Exercises

1. Write a philosophy in which you describe who you are, where you are going, and what you hope to accomplish. This philosophy should include your goals for life, your basic values, your strengths and weaknesses.
2. List six areas of potential employment and explain briefly the benefits of each.
3. Assuming you have been informed of a dental assistant position by one of the sources discussed in the chapter, write a letter of application for this position. Also, prepare a resume to accompany the letter. Make a carbon copy of the letter and the resume for your personal files.
4. Assuming you have been interviewed for the position mentioned in question 3, write an appropriate follow-up letter.
5. List five assets you have to offer that you think would attract the favorable attention of a future employer.
6. What are five ways in which an application blank might attract unfavorable attention?
7. List ten questions that you might be asked to answer during an interview.

Suggested Activities

On p. 288 are suggested activities that relate to this chapter.

Bibliography

Frederick, P.M., and Kinn, M.E.: Medical office assistant, administrative and clinical, ed. 4, Philadelphia, 1974, W.B. Saunders Co.

Fulton, P.J.: General office procedures for colleges, ed. 8, Cincinnati, 1983, South-Western Publishing Co.

Hanna, J.M., Popham, E.L., and Tilton, R.S.: Secretarial procedures and administration, ed. 6, Cincinnati, 1973, South-Western Publishing Co.

Institute for Community Development and Services, Continuing Education Service: Direction—Michigan career opportunity guide, East Lansing, MI, 1975, Michigan State University.

Place, R., Hicks, C.B., and Byers, E.E.: College secretarial procedures, ed. 4, New York, 1972, McGraw-Hill Book Co.

The graduate—a handbook for leaving school, 1975, Knoxville, TN, 1975, Approach 13-30 Corp.

3 Dental Staff Management

Behavioral Objectives

The business assistant will:
- Identify types of leadership
- Determine goals and objectives for a dental practice
- Identify functions of a manager
- Identify characteristics of a good manager
- Manage interpersonal communications of staff and doctor
- Explain the purpose of an office procedural manual
- Identify components of an office procedural manual
- Describe the contents of a personnel policy in an office procedural manual
- Discuss the procedures for conducting a staff meeting
- Write a job description
- Write an advertisement for a job application
- Describe the employee selection process
- Describe new employee training and development
- Manage staff conflict

Communication is an essential element in management and becomes a vital link in establishing a meaningful relationship between you, the doctor, other members of the staff, and the patient.

The basis for all communication is the ability to understand and to be understood by another person. The relative success of a dental practice can be measured by the ability of the staff to communicate with each other and with the patient. The form that communication takes in an office may be dictated by the type of leadership in that office.

Leadership in a Dental Practice

Leadership is vital to communication in the dental office and will determine how the staff and the doctor work together and even whether goals are established. Leadership may be authoritative, free-rein, or participatory.

Authoritative leadership allows the doctor to make all the decisions as the central authority figure. The dental assistants are not involved in any decision-making and are told only what they may or may not do within the system. This atmosphere provides little incentive for staff members, since they are merely figures who carry out specific orders. This is an efficient system, requiring less time than the other methods, but human relations researchers look upon this system with skepticism. Although governmental and educational institutions often use this system, it should be used with caution in a health care delivery system such as a dental practice. The doctor in this system generally seeks to hire dental personnel who are passive, lack a desire to make judgments, and have fewer capabilities. In an authoritative system, there is little opportunity for communication in the office, since the doctor seldom listens to the staff's ideas or considers their needs.

Free-rein leadership does not place the responsibility on any one person. The easy-going doctor does not provide direction for the staff and everyone just seems to flow along with the current. The doctor is not consistent in policies and procedures and may make erratic changes in schedules. The staff always seems to do its work, although no new techniques are ever attempted since they prefer to do their jobs in the same old way (why change?!). This doctor will probably hire assistants who are dependable and often dominant to overshadow his lack of leadership, or persons may be hired who do not enjoy challenges in their daily routine. Generally communication in this system is not definitive, because little effort is made to develop understanding among staff members. Often this type of management exists because of poor coordination and a lack of goals.

Participatory leadership is considered to have the greatest advantages for a dental practice. This form of management recognizes each member of the staff as a person whose skills are necessary in obtaining the ultimate goals for the practice. Participatory management requires that all staff members have a part in making decisions and requires the doctor be genuinely interested in the staff. The staff is required to share in the responsibility and decision-making. Therefore, such an office will include employees who are eager to accept responsibility, willing to make decisions, and seeking challenges in their daily work. This system provides an opportunity for communication, since each person seeks to understand the other person and members are encouraged to express their ideas.

Establishing Goals and Objectives

Prior to opening a dental practice the doctor should have defined a practice philosophy and established specific objectives for the practice. The lack of goals and objectives results in lack of direction for the dentist and staff and may result in poor patient relationships. As the practice grows, these goals and objectives will need to be revised. It is vital that the doctor seek input from the staff when establishing these objectives.

A common sequence for establishing objectives includes the following steps:

Develop a Practice Philosophy. The dentist identifies in a broad statement his basic concepts about patient care, business management, auxiliary utilization, and continuing education for the practice.

Develop Practice Objectives. In this stage each of the broad goals is broken into a series of specific objectives for the practice. These specific statements should be made in positive action statements that will indicate results expected to be achieved in the practice.

Develop Practice Policies. These are statements of basic policy that will affect both staff and patients. These statements may be covered by broad headings, followed by specific policies. It is wise to share these with the patients as shown in the Office Policy in Chapter 4 and with the staff as shown in the Procedural Manual in this chapter.

Develop Procedural Policies. Each of the broad statements can again be broken into specific objectives and further defined into specific tasks for all of the common office procedures. A result of this effort will be most valuable when inserted in the Procedural Manual.

Develop Business Principles. These objectives place emphasis on the actual business activities of the office. Here, the doctor will outline in numeric terms the budget process for the practice and how business activities will be managed.

Develop a Practice Standard. It is necessary for the doctor to identify a quality standard that will define a self-performance level and that expected of the staff. An explanation on how this standard is to be maintained should be provided for the staff.

As a doctor and staff work through the development of objectives for the practice, you will soon realize these become rules by which the office is managed. As the practice expands and new technology is developed, it will be necessary to review and revise these goals and objectives. Most important in participatory management is the involvement of the entire dental team in the development of these objectives.

Staff Management

After several months or years, when you have gained experience in the business procedures of the dental office, you will likely be given greater responsibility in the management of the office. As the size of the dental practice increases, doctors begin to delegate more duties to the assistants. The business office is a vital area where a person may be assigned "management" or "supervisory" responsibilities. Many of these responsibilities will require decision making in areas of office arrangement and design; development of a procedural manual; setting up staff meetings, interviewing and training new staff members; and managing staff conflict. It is not feasible to provide a management course in this brief chapter, but an introduction to some of the basic management functions may stimulate the reader to seek more in-depth management information, attend seminars, or perhaps enroll in management courses.

The term *management* has many definitions, but for the dental office, it may be defined as the process of getting things accomplished with and through people, by guiding and motivating their efforts toward common objectives.

Some people may say "managers are born, not made," but it should be realized that individuals may develop their natural skills into sound management skills through experience, effort, and learning. As you advance in this position, mistakes will be made, but remember, learning comes from mistakes as well as successes.

Functions of a Manager

The basic functions of a manager in a dental office are shown in the schematic drawing Fig. 3-1. Some managers may interpret this diagram to mean that their job is "a vicious circle." It should be realized that many of these functions overlap and that the basis for each depends on planning. If sound planning is done before beginning an activity, it is less likely that you will be confronted with crisis management, which means you spend your day handling one crisis after another.

Planning consists of identifying what is to be done in the future. The goals and objectives discussed earlier are vital to planning. The business manager will have responsibilities in long-range planning as well as activities involved in daily planning.

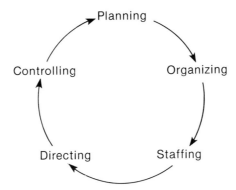

Fig. 3-1. Functions of a manager—
schematic drawing.

Organizing seeks to determine how the work will be divided and accomplished by members of the dental team. After procedures have been identified and tasks enumerated for each procedure, the business manager is required to assign the duties to specific staff members. It is absolutely essential that the doctor has given this authority to the business manager, because without this authority she cannot manage effectively.

Staffing includes the selecting, orienting, and training of employees for the office. Cooperation between the staff members will be necessary as new employees are integrated into each of the technical areas of the office. Staffing, also, involves evaluating employees, promoting them, and providing opportunities for their future development. Additionally, the business manager will be responsible for recommendations of an appropriate system of pay and benefit package.

Directing may mean issuing orders and instructions for tasks that are to be done. However, in a dental office, directing should be done in a manner that will achieve the maximum potential of the employee by guiding, teaching, and positively motivating each person to be a productive member of the dental team.

Controlling is the function of management that deals with determining whether or not the plans are being achieved and when necessary, making decisions to alter the plans in order to achieve the specific objective.

Characteristics of a Good Manager

The attitude of the business manager will have a significant influence on the staff. The following suggestions may serve to identify some of the characteristics a business manager should seek to achieve.

Be a Good Listener. Look at the person, don't stare; ask questions; restate the ideas to be sure you understand the person's message.

Utilize Feedback. Recognize nonverbal cues; use feedback as a positive source of communication; transmit feedback between management and staff.

Involve the Staff in Decision Making. Gather facts and analyze problems; develop alternatives; brainstorm with staff members; evaluate results of decision making.

Delegate Authority. Show confidence in the staff by allowing them to assume responsibility; provide freedom for them to work.

Identify Constraints Within Which Work Must Be Done. Establish time limits on production needs; allow staff to develop their own approaches within the framework you have defined.

Exercise Self Control. Emotional outbursts don't lead to constructive management; don't "talk down" to staff members.

Make Time Available to Staff. Don't be too busy to listen to a staff person; this doesn't mean you have to drop everything to listen, but make time available for staff input.

Avoid Unnecessary Delays in Decision Making. Sound decisions should be made as soon as possible; if conflicts go unresolved, greater problems may be created.

Staff Communication

Communication with staff members is in many ways like communicating with patients. You are transmitting information and understanding to another person. The difference in this communication is that the status of the persons involved has changed and the channels of communication may be more complex.

CHANNELS OF COMMUNICATION

As a dental practice increases in size, the channels of communication become more complicated. Formal and informal communication exist. A formal communication channel is dictated by the type of management that exists in the practice. Formal communication may be downward, upward, or horizontal.

Downward communication is exemplified when a doctor issues an order or mandate that is disseminated to the staff member at the next level. The basic channel is shown in Fig. 3-2. A more complex system, as shown in Fig. 3-3, illustrates an office as it increases in staff size, including several doctors and auxiliaries. Downward communication includes instructions, explanations, and communication that will aid the employee in performing work.

Fig. 3-2. Downward communication as exemplified in a traditional dental practice.

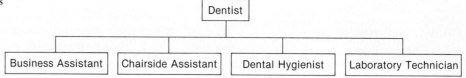

Fig. 3-3. Downward communication shown in an organizational chart of a group practice. Note—the levels of the doctors may vary according to the organization of the practice.

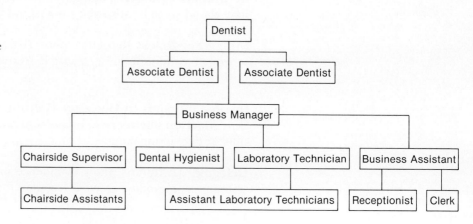

Upward channels of communication are vitally important in a formal setting. Employees should be free to communicate attitudes and feelings. This type of communication reverses the flow of information in Figs. 3-2 and 3-3 and is generally of a reporting nature and may include suggestions, complaints, or grievances. A lack of upward communication may result in dissatisfied employees.

Horizontal communication is essential for a larger organization. Sideward communication involves transmittal of information from one department to another. This type of communication exists within large offices, clinics, hospitals, and dental schools.

Informal channels of communication can also be referred to as the "grapevine." This form of communication is often feared by managers but, if handled effectively, can provide the manager with insight into staff emotions. Frequently, the grapevine carries rumors, personal interpretations, or distorted information. Fear often causes an active grapevine. It becomes the responsibility of the business manager to listen to the grapevine and eliminate rumors by explaining the true facts. Thus, you develop skill in handling tension created by the grapevine.

BARRIERS TO STAFF COMMUNICATION

The barriers that exist with patient communication—prejudice, poor listening, preoccupation, and impatience—all exist with the staff. Additional barriers, such as status or position, resistance to change and new ideas, or attitudes about work compound communication difficulties with coworkers. Since these barriers do exist, the business manager should never assume that the message being sent will be received as it was intended. You should be aware of potential misinterpretations and work to overcome barriers to improve channels of communication with the staff.

Periodically, the staff should evaluate its exchange of information. During a staff meeting, an agenda item might be the completion of a questionnaire that would indicate each staff member's feeling about communication.

Designing a Procedural Manual

The procedure manual is a valuable instrument in maintaining maximum efficiency in the dental office. It includes the doctor's philosophy of the practice and defines the job responsibilities for each team member. The manual also states in specific detail the technique to be implemented for each procedure, in both the business and clinical areas of the office. Although the manual should be written under the direction of the doctor, each member of the team should contribute equally in the construction of the manual to provide a total team effort.

In the outline below is a list of guidelines for subjects to be included in an office procedural manual. Basic formats for office manuals may be purchased to which inserts of the doctor's philosophy and specific duties relating to his practice are added. Fig. 3-4 illustrates one type of a manual available for purchase.

GUIDELINES FOR A PROCEDURAL MANUAL

I. Statement of purpose or objective of the manual
II. Statement of philosophy for the practice
III. Table of contents
IV. Office communications
   A. Vocabulary
   B. Telephone
   C. Reception techniques
   D. Written correspondence
   E. Patient education

V.   Staff policies
    A. Conduct
    B. Grooming and appearance
    C. Staff meetings
VI.   Employment policies
    A. Probationary period
    B. Promotion
    C. Hours of work
    D. Overtime
    E. Holidays
    F. Vacations
    G. Absences and leaves
    H. Salaries
    I. Insurance
    J. Additional benefits
    K. Termination of employment
    L. Personal telephone calls and personal mail
VII. Office records
    A. Patient records
    B. Transfer of records
    C. Accounts receivable
    D. Accounts payable
    E. Filing
VIII. Clinical procedures
    A. Emergencies
    B. Tray setups
    C. Sterilization
    D. Prescriptions
IX.   Inventory system
X.   Professional organizations

Fig. 3-4. An office manual. (Courtesy The Colwell Co.)

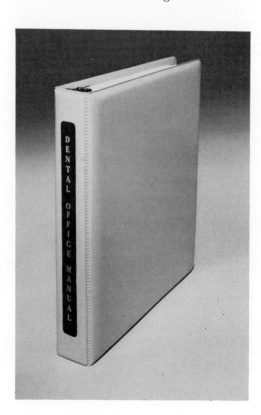

Writing a
Personnel Policy

As part of the office procedural manual, a well-defined personnel policy must be established. A fair and equitable personnel policy may help to eliminate conflicts that could arise among the team members. The boxed material below illustrates a suggested personnel policy. This policy may be altered to satisfy the needs of an individual office.

PERSONNEL POLICIES FOR THE OFFICE OF
JOSEPH W. LAKE, D.D.S.

PROBATIONARY PERIOD

Your first three months will be considered a probationary period during which Dr. Lake will see how you progress with the new work. During this period your employment may be terminated without notice.

A Merit Rating Report will be made by the doctor at the termination of the probationary period and periodically thereafter. This report is used as the basis for salary increases and promotions.

PROMOTION

Your demonstrated ability to perform your job well, your attendance and punctuality record, and your relationships with employees will all have a bearing in considering you for promotion and advancement in salary. Any outside courses of study that result in skills in addition to those already noted on your application will be added to your record to ensure complete information when reviewing your record for advancement. All employees will be reviewed every six months.

HOURS OF WORK

The basic week totals 40 working hours from 8:00 a.m. to 5:00 p.m. Monday through Friday. Lunch hour is from 12:00 p.m. to 1:00 p.m.

OVERTIME

Overtime salary is paid for units of one-half hour. Fractions of less than one-half hour of overtime are not reported. If your salary is less than $1250 a month, compensation for work authorized by the doctor in excess of 40 hours is at the rate of time and one-half beyond 40 hours in any week, or for work on Saturdays, Sundays, and holidays.

HOLIDAYS

You will have the following legal holidays with pay:

New Year's Day	Labor Day
Memorial Day	Thanksgiving
Independence Day	Christmas

When the office is closed for a religious or other holiday, announcement will be made in advance.

VACATIONS

Requests for vacation time in excess of one day must be made 30 days in advance. You will be entitled to two weeks vacation after completing twelve months of continuous employment, and four weeks vacation after ten years of employment. A legal holiday that falls within the vacation period adds one day to your vacation. Vacation salary will be paid in advance to the latest regular salary payment date falling within the vacation period.

ABSENCES AND LEAVES

Regular attendance and punctuality are necessary for the smooth functioning of the dental office, and your record in this respect will be considered in determining your advancement and salary adjustment. There are, however, certain absences that are unavoidable and for which provision will be made. In each case, Dr. Lake should be notified in advance when possible, or before 7:30 a.m. on the day of your absence. If you fail to make proper notification, the unadvised absence will be counted as absence without salary.

Continued.

PERSONNEL POLICIES FOR THE OFFICE OF
JOSEPH W. LAKE, D.D.S.—cont'd

Sick Leave for Your Own Confining Illness. (A salary will not be provided for absence due to illness of others.) When absence is for your own illness, salary is paid for up to one day for each month of employment, cumulative to 30 days. If you need sick leave in addition to the above, such a request should be made to Dr. Lake for additional time without pay.

Court Duty. If you are required to serve as a juror or witness, your absence is considered as a leave with salary.

Death in the Immediate Family. If a member of your immediate family dies, up to three days leave may be granted with salary.

Leave of Absence for Other Reasons. If you request a leave of absence for other reasons, or for a longer period than is provided with salary, various factors will be taken into consideration, including your previous work and attendance records, the length of leave you are requesting, the work needs of the office, and any other pertinent factors.

SALARIES

Payment of your salary is by check on a weekly basis, covering salary through Wednesday of the current week. Salary checks are distributed each Friday.

Salary increases are considered every six months. The quality of your work, the amount of responsibility you assume, your attendance and punctuality records, your attitude toward the staff and patients, and your length of service are factors that enter into the consideration.

Deductions from salary regularly including withholding tax and Social Security. Deductions for group insurance, hospital care, and other benefits are made only on your written request.

INSURANCE

To help provide security in times of sickness and hospitalization, health insurance is available as follows: membership in a group health insurance plan is available to all those employed up to one year on payroll deduction basis. Staff members may select this insurance at their own expense for the first twelve months of employment. Deductions for hospital care are made the first payday of each month.

At the end of twelve months, this coverage will be paid by Dr. Lake upon a successful merit rating evaluation. Coverage of your spouse and dependent children under 19 years of age may be included in your hospital care contract.

Social Security is provided through payments by you and Dr. Lake to the United States Government. Your share of the cost is deducted from each salary payment.

ADDITIONAL BENEFITS

In addition to regular salary increases, the members of the staff are eligible for several additional benefits.

Uniform Stipend. At the end of six months of successful employment, Dr. Lake will issue a uniform stipend to the Central Uniform Shop for the cost of two uniforms. At the end of twelve months an additional three uniforms will be covered. At the end of every twelve months, thereafter, a stipend for five uniforms will be issued.

Professional Organizations. At the end of twelve months of successful employment, the dues of the staff member's professional organization will be paid by Dr. Lake. The statement and proof of membership must be submitted to Dr. Lake for payment.

Education and Travel. You are encouraged to increase your skills at all times. To assure your exposure to current changes in dentistry, Dr. Lake will provide the following benefits to staff members: (1) After six months employment, payment not in excess of $150 for any educational seminar; (2) after twelve months of employment, three days absence with pay and $500 applicable to course work or educational travel; (3) after five years, five days absence and $750 applicable to course work or educational travel.

Profit Sharing. After the completion of two full years of successful employment, Dr. Lake will provide the following profit sharing bonus to each staff member: (1) 2% of total business in excess of $15,000 plus (2) 2% of total receipts in excess of $15,000.

TERMINATION OF EMPLOYMENT

Resignation. You are asked to give two weeks written notice of resignation. If you have been employed for six months or more and resign during the vacation period, having given two weeks notice, you will be compensated for your vacation according to the vacation schedule.

Release. If you are released from your position for reasons other than misconduct, in which case no notice is given, you will have notice or salary in lieu of notice as follows: If you have been employed for at least six but less than twelve months, one week; thirteen months or more, two weeks.

PERSONAL TELEPHONE CALLS AND PERSONAL MAIL

Telephone traffic is heavy at the Joseph W. Lake, D.D.S. practice. Personal telephone calls affect the work in two ways; they prohibit incoming calls from patients and they take time from your job. Limit the number of personal calls and receive incoming calls only in emergency. Similarly, the volume of mail is heavy at the office; therefore, do not use the office address for personal mail.

Preparing for a Staff Meeting

Regularly scheduled staff meetings should become a routine part of the dental practice. The staff meeting provides an opportunity to define and review the goals for the practice. Although criticism may be part of a staff meeting, such a meeting should not be designed as a gripe session. The time and length of the staff meeting will vary, according to the needs of the staff. Some offices schedule an hour per week, some close the office for one-half to a full day for a retreat session, while others find luncheon or breakfast meetings effective.

An agenda may be used in planning a staff meeting. The agenda, combined with the list of rules below, will serve to expedite the business of the staff meeting.

1. Notify each staff member of the time and place of the staff meeting. Request a return reply for attendance.
2. Determine the priority of agenda items. Obtain suggestions for these items from the staff members.
3. Provide a copy of the agenda to each staff member and adhere to the agenda items.
4. Review accomplishments.
5. Determine goals and needs for changes.
6. Establish a method for accomplishing these goals.
7. Review outcome of the meeting and provide typed minutes to the staff.
8. Maintain a strict meeting schedule.
9. Don't allow one person to monopolize the meeting.
10. Don't turn the meeting into a gripe session.

Writing a Job Description

Within the procedural manual there should be a job description for each of the positions in the office. This job description will aid you in telling prospective employees what will be expected of them on the job and will aid in training new staff members.

To write a job description you will need to do a job analysis. A job analysis involves observing the employee and gathering information about

Fig. 3-5. Job description.

Job title _____

You will report to _____

GENERAL OBJECTIVES:

The business assistant will manage the day to day activities of the business office. The maintenance of records, patients, and staff; scheduling of patients; staff interviewing/dismissal; accounts receivable and payable; inventory control; and recall will all be managed by this person.

SPECIFIC OBJECTIVES:

Maintain patient records
- Complete a clinical chart for each patient
- Maintain a financial record for each patient
- Complete insurance claim forms as needed for each patient
- Establish and maintain a recall system

Maintain an accounts receivable system using the pegboard
- Enter patient activity on the pegboard
- Maintain accounts receivable activity
- Prepare bank deposits
- Prepare statements
- Follow up insurance claims
- Follow up delinquent accounts

Perform limited accounts payable duties
- Verify invoices with monthly statements
- Write checks as directed
- Balance the bank statement
- Prepare materials for the accountant

Supervise staff personnel
- Write ads for new staff
- Conduct screening interviews
- Determine staff schedules
- Prepare for staff meeting
- Aid in staff management
- Orient new staff

Perform support duties
- Order supplies
- Establish equipment maintenance program
- Help support staff as needed

PERSONNEL REQUIREMENT:

Educational
- Certified Dental Assistant or a minimum of 5 years experience
- Knowledge of automated equipment used in the office
- Business course work
- Knowledge or experience in management

Emotional requirements
- Must be able to work with any employee and be able to resolve conflicts between employees
- Must be able to discuss all dental needs with patients, be objective, and be pleasant to them
- Must be able to cooperate with other dental office staff personnel
- Must be able to work with the doctor and convey needs to staff in a participatory manner

SALARY:

$14,500-$21,500 plus benefits
Salary based on the salary chart in the office procedure manual.

Date prepared: 1/25/-

From: Korneluk, G.N.: Job descriptions: put it in writing to put into practice, Gen. Dent., March-April, 1983.

the job. You will list the tasks that comprise the job, determine the skills, personality characteristics, and educational background needed for the employee to perform this job satisfactorily. A job description is then reviewed by the staff, revised as necessary, and placed in the procedural manual. An outline for a job description is shown in Fig. 3-5.

Writing an Advertisement

The content of an advertisement for new staff members should be the result of a well-thought-out job description. List the skills you expect the person to have, require a resume, and identify attractive features of the job, i.e., benefits, salary, working conditions. If you expect to attract highly qualified candidates, your advertisement cannot be a mundane, brief statement seeking inexperienced people. Periodically look at the classified ads in the local paper for ideas in other allied health professions. Compare the two advertisements in Figs. 2-1 and 2-2. Which advertisement presents a greater challenge for a prospective employee? The ad seeking an inexperienced person will probably get more response, but this isn't a contest. The procedure of advertising should seek to screen potential candidates. A request for an educated person cuts down on potential training costs for the doctor and can assure a minimal level of education.

Interviewing Prospective Employees

Part of the management role for the business assistant may be interviewing applicants for a position on the staff. This is an important responsibility and requires a great deal of skill. The following suggestions may aid you when conducting an interview.
1. Have a well-defined job description.
2. Have the applicant complete a job application.
3. Determine the competencies required to fulfill this job.
4. Determine how you will measure an applicant's ability. In some instances, tests may be utilized to measure certain abilities, such as typing speed and accuracy.
5. Investigate references the applicant has provided. This confirms the accuracy of an applicant's statements.
6. Explain the requirements of the job completely.
7. Determine key questions to ask in the interview. Gain confidence in questioning the applicant to reflect each facet of the individual's background. Ask such questions as, "Tell me about your previous job experiences." "What is your attitude toward your previous working experience?" "What do you feel your strengths and weaknesses are for the position available in this office?"
8. Review your feelings toward the applicant. Were you comfortable? Was the applicant an active participant in the conversation? Was the individual either shy or domineering?
9. Make accurate observations about the applicant's answers, grammar, and nonverbal cues during the interview. Use a check-off form to assure each candidate is evaluated on the same basis. Record evaluations as soon as the interview is completed to assure you don't forget the responses.

The applicant should have the opportunity to tour the office. This is a good time, if convenient, for the rest of the staff to meet the candidate. Inform the applicant of the plans for arriving at a decision and a date by which the decision will be made.

Once all of the candidates have been interviewed and the decision made about each, the person to be hired should be contacted promptly. A letter of confirmation should be sent to the new employee stating the conditions of employment, i.e., wages, hours, promotions, beginning date, and other conditions agreed upon during previous discussions. Probationary periods should be identified in the letter which allows either party to terminate employment within an established period of time, without fear of penalty. It is wise to have the employee sign the letter and a copy is then retained by the employee and a copy is placed in the employee file. A letter should also be sent to candidates not being hired and their applications may remain on file if desired.

New Employee Training

A well-organized procedural manual will provide smooth transition for the new employee into the practice. Time for the new employee to become well established in the office will vary according to the individual office. Among the many activities involved in new employee training, you should be able to:

1. Describe how the practice is run and what standards are required of the staff.
2. Explain the organizational chart and job descriptions.
3. Complete employee documents, i.e., federal and state tax forms.
4. Review procedural techniques.
5. Allow time for observation but let the skills and responsibilities of the new employee be utilized as soon as possible.
6. Identify areas of strengths and weaknesses. Positive reinforcement is necessary to create confidence. However, poor performance should be altered to avoid reinforcement of less than quality work. It is easier to correct poor performance early in training than later when it seriously affects the office production.
7. Provide additional training beyond the educational experiences already achieved. This may be accomplished within the office or may require a more formal setting in a nearby school.
8. Evaluate the performance of the new employee regularly. This allows changes to be made in performance and provides the staff person with knowledge of their status.
9. Review progress with adequate promotion via benefits or a pay increase.
10. Terminate an employee if substandard performance continues. If all efforts to improve the employee's performance have failed, it is wise to terminate the employee promptly rather than to continue with substandard performance.

Managing Conflict

Some business managers become defensive and irritated when confronted with a complaint. Some individuals feel that a complaint is a reflection on them personally. However, conflicts are a normal function between a manager and an employee, or between the patient and a member of the staff. Concern should be raised if numerous complaints arise, since this may indicate a serious problem.

Regardless of the nature of the complaint, the business manager should review the details of the complaint and seek to resolve the problem quickly. Steps in resolving the problem might include the following:

1. **Make time available** as soon as possible to discuss the problem. A delay may result in additional conflict or may be interpreted that you are not interested in listening to the problem.
2. **Listen patiently** to all the issues, keeping an open mind. You can gain confidence of the staff member if you encourage the person to talk and if you indicate you want to provide fair treatment.

3. **Determine the real issue.** Frequently, a complaint is made about a problem, when in reality, a deeper concern is the real issue. For example, a person may be complaining about unfair work assignments, when actually, a personality clash may exist between two staff members.

4. **Exercise self control.** Avoid arguments or personality conflicts between the complaining parties. Emotional outbursts generally do not lead to contructive resolution of the problem. Should this result, it is wise to terminate the meeting until a future meeting can be scheduled when the problem can be discussed in a calm manner.

5. **Avoid a delay in decision making.** A dental office is a relatively small business organization and allowing a conflict to go unresolved can cause undue stress on the entire staff. If it is necessary to delay a decision, let the persons involved know the status of the problem.

6. **Maintain a record.** Documentation of meetings or discussions are helpful should future conflict arise over the same problem. It is impossible for you to recall all of the issues about an incident. Therefore, information should be retained in the employee file or appropriate area for future reference.

It is not easy to resolve conflict. Most of us wish to avoid it. However, we must realize conflict will arise whenever we have two or more people working together. As a business manager, you should try to be fair and objective. If you follow the suggestions listed earlier, you will have at least attempted to resolve the complaint in a professional manner and will possibly avoid minor conflicts that can escalate into major crises.

Exercises

1. Explain the three types of leadership that might be found in a dental office. Reflect on offices that you have visited and identify the leadership style of each doctor. What effect does leadership have on communication in each of these offices?

2. Write a job description for a chairside assistant, business assistant, and dental hygienist. What tasks will be identified for each of these jobs in a job analysis?

3. Review classified advertisements in a local paper. Compare the content of ads in various health occupations. What characteristics appeal to you in these ads? Why?

4. Using the job analysis from Question 2, write a classified advertisement for each job. Hint: It might be beneficial to do this as a group activity and share advertisements. Which ads would be most appealing? Which ads would be more specific and limit responses to desired candidates?

5. How would you handle these conflict situations?
   a. Dr. Lake reprimands you for having forgotten to make a telephone call he requested you to make. What would you do?
   b. A chairside assistant in the office criticizes another assistant to you for wearing bizarre jewelry. What would be your response?
   c. Office hours in an office for the staff are 8:15 AM to 5:00 PM. An assistant is chronically late, arriving 15 to 20 minutes after the assigned time each day. She always leaves by 5:00 PM and seldom is late leaving for lunch. Friction is occurring among the staff. The doctor doesn't seem to be concerned. Is this really a problem? What are the issues involved here? Can there be a resolution? What action should be taken? Who should take the action?

Bibliography

Byars, L.L., and Rue, L.W.: Personnel management: concepts and applications, Philadelphia, 1979, W.B. Saunders Co.

Chapman, E.N.: Your attitude is showing—a primer on human relations, Palo Alto CA, 1971, Science Research Associates, Inc.

Cutler, M.: Office design: key to your professional image, Dent. Manag., Oct., 1975, pp. 36-56.

Fulton, P.J.: General office procedures for colleges, ed. 8, Cincinnati, 1983, South-Western Publishing Co.

Gossett, D.G.: Design + equipment + communication = efficiency, Dent. Survey **51**(5):80-82, 1975.

Haimann, T., and Hilgert, R.: Supervision: concepts and practices of management, ed. 3, Cincinnati, 1982, South-Western Publishing Co.

PA Ideas: Staff meetings that get things done, Professional Budget Plan, Madison, WI, Form #0158 873 10M (a pamphlet).

PA Ideas: The shape of the interview, Professional Budget Plan, Madison, WI, Form #0 222 575 5M (a pamphlet).

good hunting, I'd do it, too. I had forgotten how *predatory* English females can be!"

As an English female, Francesca thought it her duty to take public exception to such a generalization, even though she tended to agree with the assessment much of the time. Had he thought her predatory five years ago? Was that why he went away so quickly, no doubt in disgust of her? "Really, my lord—" she began her defense of her sex.

"Oh, you needn't worry. I didn't mean you. I know only too well that *you* have no designs on me, my lady. It is why I have particularly sought you out. I must breathe for a moment before one more young lady tries to flirt with me." And so saying, he threw himself into a chair beside her, or came as close to doing so as a pair of tight-fitting pantaloons, a strict upbringing, and a very elegant drawing room would allow.

"Well, old man," said Mr. Symington, rising to his full lanky six-feet-plus, "if you plan to leave the field open to us lesser mortals for a moment, I'll just go say a word to Miss Hollys. You know, Dev, if you really wanted to give the rest of us fellows a break, you'd adjourn immediately to the billiard room. Out of sight, out of mind, y'know." And sketching a grinning bow to Francesca, he crossed the room to the most current object of his affections.

"Are you so certain that I shall not try to flirt with you, my lord?" asked Francesca. "Such a very *eligible* and *interesting* gentleman must certainly be a temptation," she finished with a nice blend of archness and sweetness and a maidenly flutter of her golden lashes.

"Don't you dare to! I shall not be responsible for my actions if you do," he answered in mock, but only slightly mock, horror. "But I have no fear of it. I know I shall be safe with you." The elaborate casualness with which he spoke struck her as not quite true. Did it hide a note of bitterness? And whatever did he mean, anyway?

It had, after all, been he who had abandoned her five years ago.

"Oh, yes, my lord," she said. "Quite safe."

His blue eyes darkened at her tone. He wondered what he could have said to upset her. "I do wish you would put away all this 'my lord' business. I am quite unused to it—no one lordships anyone in America, you know—and I am finding it wearying in the extreme. My friends call me Devlin."

"Am I to take that as an offer of friendship . . . Devlin?"

"Of course. A friend is merely the opposite of an enemy, and I hope we are not that, my lady."

"I see no reason why we should be," she replied coolly, much more coolly than she felt. "And my name is Francesca."

"It suits you, you know, in its regalness. Makes you sound like some cool Italian beauty sitting on the balcony of her palazzo and gazing placidly down onto a Venetian piazza, wondering at the robust antics of the throngs below."

She could not keep a gasp of surprise from her lips. Was that really how he saw her? She could not know that he had only this evening been told of the nicknames bestowed on her by the unlucky London bucks she had spurned. "The Ice Goddess" and "The Citadel" were two of the more common. They had replaced "Carefree Cesca," which had graced her just three or four years earlier.

"I should hope I am not so far removed from life as that, Devlin. To merely look down upon it like it was a play on a stage." The words rang hollow in her own ears, for was that not precisely how she had been viewing herself of late, the very reason her life had been so empty?

"I should hope so too, Francesca," he said quietly, remembering a bright-eyed, eager girl with a woman's passions, and wondering where she had gone. "I should hope so too."

Eyes may say much, but the gaze of these two locked on each other had time to murmur little more than a word before the ripple of laughter that was the calling card of Roxanna Gordon joined in the conversation. "Naughty Cesca!" she chided. "Monopolizing the only truly interesting man present. I have brought you more tea, Devlin, though I don't imagine you can bear the wishy-washy stuff. I imagine you frontiersmen stick with rum or brandy or some such delightfully masculine drink."

"Whiskey, Mrs. Gordon," he replied, slipping easily into a bantering tone. "And on occasion coffee, but coffee such as you have never tasted, I'm sure. Roasted black as coal and brewed just as strong. It's thick and hot and chewy. A bit of heaven, in fact. I don't advise it for a lady, however," he continued mischievously. "The Americans are fond of saying it will put hair on your chest."

"Oh la!" she cried on a ripple of mirth, and tapped his hand with her busily working fan. "How naughty you are!" She had long since lost the ability to blush on command, to her vast annoyance, and needs must use her sultry smile instead. She gave him one of her best. "And you, Devlin? Can you prove the aphorism a true one? I daresay you can, but how intriguing to wonder in uncertainty."

Disgusted at the woman's forwardness, though she had been rather amused by it in the past, Francesca excused herself and went to where Sarah was pouring out fresh tea. Devlin was left to suffer alone the pointed flirtations of Mrs. Gordon.

Luckily for his lordship, the beginning of hunting on the morrow precluded a late night. Everyone was eager to be well-rested and in good trim for the opening meet. It was not long, therefore, before Sarah led the ladies up

the stairs to their bedchambers. The gentlemen followed
very shortly.

The stars glittered, and the dew fell. The Stopper-up
rode over the fields filling foxholes in preparation for the
festivities to come. The dogs snoozed peacefully, as yet
unaware of the excitement the morning would bring.

The lights of Hockleigh winked out one by one until
the great house lay in darkness, gilded only by the soft
glow of the moon as it slid lower in the sky.

Lady Francesca slept.